HEALING THROUGH WORDS

1000 Positive Affirmations Book

for
Health, Success, Wealth, Love,
Happiness, Fitness, Weight Loss,
Self Esteem, Confidence, Sleep,
Healing, Abundance, Motivational
Quotes, and Much More!

love

hope

believe

dream

INTRODUCTION

Affirmations are positive statements that can help you to challenge and overcome self-sabotaging and negative thoughts. When you repeat them often, and believe in them, you can start to make positive changes.

You might consider affirmations to be unrealistic "wishful thinking." But try looking at positive affirmations this way: many of us do repetitive exercises to improve our physical health, and affirmations are like exercises for our mind and outlook. These positive mental repetitions can reprogram our thinking patterns so that, over time, we begin to think – and act – differently.

The benefits of Affirmations are endless, they have helped a multitude of people all over the world achieve great things, but more importantly, they can help you make positive changes in your life.

Affirmations have the power to motivate you to act on certain things, help you to concentrate on achieving your goals in life, give you the power to change your negative thinking patterns and replace them with positive thinking patterns, assist you in accessing a new belief system, but above all, affirmations can reaffirm the positivity back into your life and help regain or increase your self-confidence.

For Affirmations to truly work, you need to repeat the affirmation daily, and truly believe in the words you are saying. For example "I will not compare myself to others." Now that is an affirmation that is targeted to boost your self-confidence and your own self-worth, but you need to believe in that statement and repeat it 3 to 5 times a day.

Affirmations are a powerful and life-changing tool, use them wisely.

We always love to offer free books to our readers.

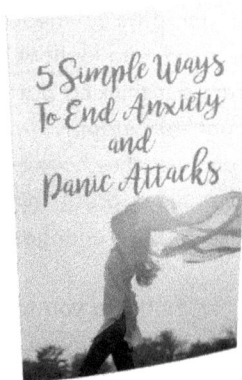

5 Simple Ways To End Anxiety and Panic Attacks

Get your free book by scanning the **QR** code or by sending an email to the address bellow.

 Catherine.Worren@yahoo.com

I CAN WITHSTAND ADVERSITY AND COME OUT STRONGER THAN EVER.

I AM WORTHY OF MORE THAN I REALIZE.

I AM A GREAT SISTER, EVEN WHEN I FEEL AS THOUGH I DON'T DESERVE THAT TITLE.

I CAN DO ANYTHING I PUT MY MIND TO.

I AM UNIQUE.

I CAN DO GREAT THINGS IF I PUT MY MIND TO IT.

I AM A BEAUTIFUL SOUL.

I AM CAPABLE.

I CAN DO MORE THAN I EVER IMAGINED POSSIBLE.

I DESERVE THE GOOD.

I AM ONE OF A KIND.

I DO NOT NEED OTHERS TO MAKE ME CONTENT.

WHEN I DREAM, I WAKE UP AFTER AND FIND REALITY IS JUST AS GOOD.

I CAN BE GOOFY AND QUIRKY.
NOTHING GETS ME DOWN.

I WILL INSPIRE THE WORLD WITH MY WORDS. I AM
FIERCE.

I WILL CHANGE THE WAY I PUT MYSELF
DOWN.

I WILL LET GO OF INSECURITIES.

BREATHING IN AND OUT;

I WILL LET OUT THE OLD AIR AND BECKON IN THE NEW.

SELF-LOVE IS EVERYTHING.

SELF-LOVE IS LEARNING TO LOVE DESPITE ALL THE
THINGS YOU'VE NEVER LIKED
ABOUT YOURSELF.

WE MUST ACCEPT WHO WE ARE
TO BECOME THE VERSION OF OURSELVES
WE HOPE TO BE.

WHEN I DANCE, I MOVE TO THE RHYTHM OF MY SOUL.

I AM DRIVEN BY THE DETERMINATION I HAVE WITHIN MYSELF.

I AM THE ONLY PERSON I NEED.

I CAN FIND THE LIGHT IN ANY SITUATION.

I AM POSITIVE.

MY ENERGY DRAWLS PEOPLE IN.

I AM A PASSIONATE PERSON.

I AM A LIFELONG LEARNER.

NOW IS THE MOMENT TO SEIZE.

TAKE ADVANTAGE OF EVERY OPPORTUNITY, YOU NEVER KNOW WHEN IT WILL BE OVER.

I AM GRATEFUL FOR THE EXPERIENCES THAT HAVE BROUGHT ME TO WHERE I AM NOW.

I AM A WARRIOR.

STRONG DOESN'T BEGIN TO COVER WHAT I AM.

I FIGHT FOR WHAT I WANT.

I DON'T GET DISCOURAGED, INSTEAD, I SAY, "NEXT TIME."

I CAN STAND UP FOR MYSELF.

I HAVE THE POWER TO CREATE REAL CHANGE.

I AM WORTHY OF LOVE AND WARMTH.

I CAN MAKE THE WORLD A BETTER PLACE.

I CAN TEACH MYSELF TO TAKE IT DAY BY DAY.

I AM CAPABLE OF AMAZING THINGS THAT NO ONE WOULD'VE EXPECTED.

I AM GENUINE IN ALL THINGS.

I STAY LOYAL TO MY PARTNERS.

I GIVE THE LOVE I HOPE TO RECEIVE.

I AM A GIVING PERSON.

SEEING OTHERS HAPPY, WARMS MY HEART.

I THRIVE OFF THE ENERGY OF OTHER PEOPLE.

I NEED POSITIVE ENERGY AROUND ME TO PUSH FORWARD IN THE DARKNESS.

I KNOW MY WORTH.

I CAN BUST OUT WORK AND GET STUFF DONE.

WORK CAN'T GET ME DOWN.

INSTEAD OF GIVING INTO OTHERS, I STAND FOR MY VALUES ALWAYS.

I AM JOYFUL.

I AM RADIANT.

WHEN I SMILE, PEOPLE AROUND ME FOLLOW SUIT.

I GLOW WHEN I AM HAPPY.

I AM A BRILLIANT MIND.

GLOWING: I AM HAPPINESS MANIFEST.

I AM BEAUTIFUL.

I AM BEAUTIFUL BUT THAT DOES NOT DEFINE ME.

I AM ALLURING.

FLIRTY AND MISCHIEVOUS, I AM FUN TO BE AROUND.

I AM CHARMING.

PEOPLE OFTEN SAY AFTER MEETING ME, THAT I PUT MY "CHARM" ON THEM.

I AM DELIGHTFUL.
LIKE THE SUN, I SHINE AND CAST MY LIGHT OVER OTHERS.

I AM NOT AFRAID, BECAUSE I AM IN CONTROL OF MY JOURNEY.

I AM A POSITIVE FORCE OF GOOD.

I AM A GREAT ROLE MODEL FOR OTHER WOMEN.

I AM A SUCCESS STORY.

MY FAMILY SHOULD BE PROUD OF WHO I HAVE BECOME.

WHEN THINGS GET HARD, I DO NOT WAIVER. I KEEP WORKING EVEN WHEN THINGS GET HARD.

I AM PERSISTENT AND I GET THINGS DONE.

NOTHING CAN STOP ME FROM ACCOMPLISHING MY GOALS.

EVERY DAY I SHOULD LOOK IN THE MIRROR AND TELL MYSELF I AM A QUEEN.

I CAN BE PRODUCTIVE IF I TRY HARD ENOUGH.

I WON'T LET OTHER PEOPLE GET ME DOWN.

I DON'T LET OTHER PEOPLE'S OPINIONS OF ME GET ME DOWN.

YOU ARE A SHINING STAR.

YOU ARE WHAT DREAMS ARE MADE OF.

NOTHING CAN STOP YOU.

YOU CAN ONLY GO UP FROM HERE.

YOU ARE GROWING LIKE THE QUICKENING HUES OF EVERY SEASON.

LIKE FALL YOU WILL CHANGE YOUR SURROUNDINGS AND MAKE WAY FOR FLOURISHING.

YOU ARE BEAUTY AND GRACE AND LIGHT AND LAUGHTER AND WARMTH.

PEOPLE LOVE BEING AROUND YOU.

YOUR VOICE IS MUSIC TO EARS.

IF THE YOUNGER VERSION OF YOU, COULD SEE
WHERE YOU ARE RIGHT NOW, THEY'D BE PROUD.

EVERY DAY THAT YOU DECIDE YOU ARE WORTHY OF
LOVE, OTHERS WILL NOTICE.

I GET BETTER EVERY DAY.

WHEN I TRY MY HARDEST, NOTHING CAN STOP ME.

I AM A ROLE MODEL.

I AM STRENGTH MANIFESTED.

I AM WARMTH MANIFESTED.

I AM LIGHT MANIFESTED.

I AM JOY MANIFESTED.

I AM HAPPINESS MANIFESTED.

I AM POSITIVITY MANIFESTED.

I AM CONFIDENCE MANIFESTED.

I AM RADIANCE MANIFESTED.

I AM KIND.

I AM TRUTHFUL.

I AM TRUE TO MY WORD.

I MAKE THE MOST OF EVERY SITUATION.

I AM A SURVIVOR.

I AM WORTH THE TIME AND EFFORT I SPEND ON MY
SELF-CARE.

I CAN BE HONEST ABOUT HOW I'M FEELING.

I CAN TAKE BREAKS WHEN NECESSARY.

I KNOW HOW MUCH FOR MYSELF IS TOO MUCH.

I CAN WORK ON MY BAD HABITS AND REVERSE THEM.

I CAN HEAL FROM THE BAD THINGS THAT HAVE
HAPPENED TO ME.

I CAN BE A BETTER PERSON FOR OTHERS.

I AM A GREAT FRIEND.

I AM DESERVING OF THE LOVE I GIVE OUT.

I AM AN INTELLIGENT BEING.

I RADIATE CALM.

PEOPLE FEEL PEACEFUL WHEN THEY ARE IN MY PRESENCE.

I KNOW HOW TO FIND THE BRIGHT SIDE.

MY GLASS IS ALWAYS HALF FULL.

I CAN FIND THE POSITIVES IN EVERY SITUATION.

I KNOW WHAT IT'S LIKE TO BE HURT, SO I TRY NOT TO HURT OTHERS.

I AM WORTHY OF SO MUCH LOVE.

I FEEL CONTENT RIGHT NOW, IN THIS MOMENT AND THE NEXT.

I AM DESERVING OF JOY.

I HAVE EVERYTHING I NEED.

MY BODY IS A VESSEL AND I TAKE CARE OF IT AS BEST AS I CAN.

I NURTURE MY BODY.

I WORK ON HEALING MY INNER PAIN.

I AM SELFLESS AND KIND.

I TAKE TIME FOR MYSELF. I KNOW I AM WORTH IT.

MUSIC SPEAKS TO MY SOUL.

I WORK ON HEALING MY INNER CHILD.

I AM DESERVING OF THE LOVE I WANT.

I AM DESERVING OF A PARTNER THAT LOVES ME FOR ME.

I HAVE MADE IT SO FAR.

I AM PROUD OF MYSELF.

I AM PROUD TO BE A WOMAN.

I AM ENOUGH.

I AM ENOUGH FOR MYSELF.

I AM ENOUGH FOR OTHER PEOPLE.

I HELP PEOPLE AS OFTEN AS I CAN.

I SEIZE THE MOMENT.

I SEIZE EVERY MOMENT AND TRY NOT TO WASTE TIME.

I KNOW WHAT I AM CAPABLE OF, AND NO ONE CAN
HOLD ME BACK.

I AM A PRESENT AND THOUGHTFUL PERSON.

I TURN MY PHONE OFF AND ENJOY CONNECTING WITH
OTHERS IN PERSON.

COMMUNICATION COMES EASILY TO ME.

I AM GREAT AT HOLDING CONVERSATIONS.

I AM FUNNY.

PEOPLE ENJOY TALKING TO ME.

I AM OUTGOING.

I DON'T LET THE ANXIETY OF MESSING UP GET TO ME.

I AM A PRODUCTIVE PERSON.

I FEEL GOOD.

EVERYTHING I NEED IS WITHIN ME.

I AM TRUE TO MYSELF 100% OF THE TIME.

I NOURISH MY BODY.

I KNOW THE FUTURE WILL BE WORTH WAITING FOR.

I HAVE HOPE THAT THINGS WILL GET BETTER IN TIME.

I DON'T WORRY OR STRESS; I CHOSE TO RELAX AND
ENJOY THE PROCESS.

LIFE CANNOT GET ME DOWN.

I LOVE ROLLERCOASTERS; THAT'S WHAT LIFE IS.

EVERY MOMENT SPENT DOING THE THINGS I LOVE IS A
MOMENT SPENT WELL.

I AM PASSION AND SOUL.

WHEN I HAVE SELF-DOUBT, I REMIND
MYSELF THAT I AM WORTHY OF MORE THAN MY
INSECURITIES WILL LET ME BELIEVE.

I DON'T NEED OTHERS TO MAKE ME HAPPY.

I DON'T NEED MONEY OR CLOTHES TO BE CONTENT.

I AM HAPPY WITHOUT THE MATERIAL THINGS IN MY LIFE.

I AM NOT A MATERIAL GIRL.

I DO NOT NEED TO SPEND MONEY TO FEEL JOY.

I AM GOOD AT SAVING.

I CAN SAVE FOR LONG PERIODS OF TIME AND WORK
TOWARDS LONG-TERM GOALS.

I AM A MONEY-SAVER.

MONEY DOESN'T DRIVE ME.

I AM DRIVEN BY MY WANT TO SUCCEED.

I AM DRIVEN BY LOVE.

I AM DRIVEN BY LIGHT AND GOODNESS.

I WANT TO DO GOOD FOR PEOPLE.

I WANT TO HELP OTHERS.

I WANT TO LEAVE THE WORLD A BETTER PLACE FOR
THE NEXT GENERATION.

I DANCE TO MY OWN BEAT.

I AM ONE OF A KIND, A GEMSTONE UNCOVERED.

I UNDERSTAND HOW IMPORTANT IT IS TO KEEP LEARNING.

I HAVE FAITH IN HUMANITY.

I HAVE THE BEST INTEREST OF OTHERS IN MIND, ALWAYS.

I AM OPEN TO SEEING OTHER PERSPECTIVES.

I AM OPEN TO CHANGING MY MIND.

EVERYTHING THAT HAPPENS IS FROM NOW ON.

PEOPLE CAN FEEL SAFE WITH ME.

I MAKE THE BEST OF EVERY MOMENT AND SITUATION.

I KNOW HOW TO MAKE THE MOST OF LIFE.

I UNDERSTAND I DON'T KNOW EVERYTHING AND THAT IS OK.

I'M LEARNING HOW TO BE THE BEST VERSION OF MYSELF.

EVERY DAY IS A NEW DAY TO BE HAPPY.

EVERY DAY IS A NEW DAY TO BE THE BEST VERSION OF MYSELF.

EVERY DAY IS A CHANCE TO START ANEW.

YOU DON'T HAVE TO BE PERFECT TO BE VALID.

YOU ARE IN CONTROL OF YOUR FUTURE; NO ONE ELSE.

YOU ARE MAGNIFICENT.

DON'T LET ANYONE STEAL YOUR LIGHT.

YOU ARE BEAUTY AND LIGHT.

YOU ARE EVERYTHING.

YOU ARE THE REASON SOMEONE SMILES.

YOU CAN DO ANYTHING, BE ANYTHING.

THE SKY IS LIMITLESS FOR YOU.

GO OUT AND LIVE IN THE MOMENT.

I DON'T CARE ABOUT WHAT OTHERS THINK. I CHOOSE
NOT TO CARE ABOUT WHAT OTHERS THINK OF ME.

MY SOUL SINGS TO ITS OWN SONG.

I AM BEAUTIFULLY UNIQUE.

OTHERS DON'T GET ME DOWN, I AM UNSTOPPABLE.
I KNOW MY PASSION AND I LET IT WORK THROUGH ME.

I AM ENOUGH FOR MYSELF AND SOMEONE ELSE.

I AM WORTHY OF GREAT THINGS.

I ATTRACT AMAZING THINGS.

I ATTRACT THE LOVE I DESERVE.

I ATTRACT LIGHT AND GOODNESS.

I ATTRACT THE BEST IN LIFE.

I AM GRATEFUL FOR EVERYTHING I HAVE I AM
GRATEFUL FOR THE LITTLE THINGS.

I AM GRATEFUL FOR MUSIC.

I AM GRATEFUL FOR LAUGHTER.

I AM GRATEFUL FOR MY FAMILY & LOVED ONES.

I AM GRATEFUL FOR THE DAYS SPENT RELAXING
BECAUSE I KNOW I DESERVE TO REST.

TODAY IS A GREAT DAY TO BE ALIVE.

I AM GRATEFUL FOR LIFE.

I AM GRATEFUL FOR THE EARTH AND NATURE.

I FEEL CONNECTED TO THE NATURAL WORLD.

I FEEL AT PEACE WITH MYSELF.

I FEEL AT PEACE WITH MY LIFE.

I FEEL HAPPY ABOUT WHERE I AM RIGHT NOW.

I'M STILL GROWING, EVERY DAY.

I WANT TO BE A GREAT FRIEND AND CONFIDANT.

I WANT TO HELP PEOPLE EXPLORE THEIR PASSION IN LIFE.

I WANT TO GUIDE SOMEONE IN THEIR JOURNEY.

I WANT TO BE A HELPING HAND TO THOSE WHO NEED IT.

I AM KIND.

I AM COMPASSIONATE.

I AM EMPATHETIC.

I AM A GREAT PERSON.

I CAN'T POSSIBLY COMPARE MY STORY TO ANYONE ELSE'S.

I KNOW WHERE I AM SUPPOSED TO BE.

I CAN RELAX KNOWING EVERYTHING IS GOING TO BE OK.

EVERYTHING IS GOING TO BE FINE.

I HELP MY FAMILY WHEN THEY NEED ME.

I AM EXCITED BY THE SMALLEST THINGS.

I AM EXCITED TO GO OUT AND LIVE.

I WANT TO EXPERIENCE EVERYTHING I POSSIBLY CAN
IN LIFE.

I AM EXCITED TO INSPIRE THE NEXT GENERATIONS.

I AM EXCITED TO GET UP EVERY DAY.

THE QUIET MOMENTS IN LIFE ARE EVERYTHING.

I KNOW WHAT IT'S LIKE TO BE ISOLATED, SO I TRY TO
CONNECT WITH PEOPLE WHO SEEM LONELY.

I DO NOT DWELL ON THE PAST.

I DO NOT OVERTHINK MY JOURNEY.

I DO NOT LIVE IN THE PAST.

I LOOK FORWARD TO MY FUTURE AND SAY "ONWARD!"

I DO NOT DWELL ON THE NEGATIVE THINGS IN LIFE.

I KNOW MYSELF BETTER THAN ANYONE
ELSE.

I AM A TALENTED INDIVIDUAL. I USE MY SKILLS IN LIFE!

I KNOW WHERE I AM TODAY IS A DIRECT PRODUCT OF
THE HARD WORK I'VE PUT IN.

I AM DESERVING OF SELF-LOVE AND AFFIRMATION.

I DON'T LET ANY BEAUTY STANDARDS CHANGE THE
WAY I FEEL ABOUT MY WEIGHT.

I DON'T LET THIN CULTURE AFFECT MY EATING HABITS.

I DON'T LET DIET CULTURE AFFECT MY
EATING HABITS.

I ACCEPT MY BODY HOW IT IS.

I ACCEPT MY ENTIRE BEING FOR HOW IT IS RIGHT
NOW.

I ACCEPT MYSELF.

I ACCEPT ALL THE THINGS I CANNOT CHANGE.

I EMBRACE THE UNKNOWN.

I EMBRACE THE CURRENT MOMENT.

I ACCEPT THE LOVE I DESERVE IN MY LIFE.

I ACCEPT THE TREATMENT I KNOW I DESERVE.

I DON'T ALLOW PEOPLE WHO HAVE HARMED ME, BACK INTO MY LIFE.

I KNOW HOW TO TELL PEOPLE TO BACK OFF WHEN NEED BE.

I AM CONFIDENT IN MY CHOICES AND DECISIONS.

I KNOW WHAT MATTERS MOST TO ME.

I CAN BE MYSELF WITHOUT FEAR OF BEING JUDGED.

I KNOW MY WORTHINESS.

I CAN LET GO OF THE HURT. AND LEAN INTO LOVE AND HEALING.

I CAN BE THE PERSON I ALWAYS HOPED TO BECOME.

I AM IN CHARGE OF MY OWN DESTINY.

I OVERSEE MY DESTINY.

I DON'T LOOK FORWARD TO A TIME FAR AWAY, I ACCEPT THE NOW, FOR ALL OF THE GREATNESS IN THE MUNDANE.

I AM A SHIP PASSING ALONG A WIDE SEA OF POSSIBILITIES.

I AM A MATCH WAITING TO BE LIT.

I HAVE A FIRE BURNING INSIDE OF ME, I HAVE BURNING ASPIRATIONS.

I AM THE MOMENT.

I AM THE TREE THAT STANDS TALL.

I AM THE TREE THAT STANDS TALL AGAINST THE SHAKING.

I DO NOT WAIVER UNDER PRESSURE.

I DO NOT GIVE IN TO THE SADNESS THAT SOMETIMES PULLS ME UNDER.

I DO NOT TAKE THINGS PERSONALLY.

I UNDERSTAND NO ONE'S JOURNEY LOOKS LIKE MINE, AND THAT'S OK.

I WORK ON MY OWN TIMELINE.

GOOD THINGS ARE WORTH WAITING FOR.

I KNOW I AM WORTH WAITING FOR.

THINGS MIGHT NOT BE GREAT TODAY, BUT
TOMORROW IS A NEW DAY.

TOMORROW IS A NEW CHANCE TO MAKE A CHANGE.
PATIENCE IS A VIRTUE I HOLD CLOSE.

I AM NOT EASILY ANGERED.

I AM NOT EASILY HURT.

I HAVE THICK SKIN, AND I DON'T TAKE OTHERS TOO
SERIOUSLY.

I CAN DECIDE WHAT PATH I TAKE IN LIFE.

IT IS NOT EASY TO GET ME DOWN.

I AM FULL OF HEART.

I UNDERSTAND THE THINGS I WANT IN LIFE ARE GOING TO REQUIRE A LOT OF WORK.

I AM WILLING TO PUT IN THE WORK IT WILL TAKE FOR ME TO SUCCEED.

I AM WILLING TO TRY THINGS THAT I'VE NEVER TRIED BEFORE.

I AM WILLING TO HEAR AN OUTSIDE PERSPECTIVE ON A PROBLEM.

I AM WILLING TO CHANGE MY OPINION ON A TOPIC.

I AM WILLING TO HEAR PEOPLE OUT.

I BELIEVE IN MY WORK. I BELIEVE IN MYSELF.

I KNOW NOTHING COMES EASY.

I KNOW THAT TO GET THE THINGS I WANT;

IT IS GOING TO TAKE A LOT OF HARD WORK. TO GET WHERE I WANT TO BE, I MUST WORK HARD.

I HAVE A GREAT WORK ETHIC.

MY WORK IS IMPORTANT TO ME.

I PUT THE EFFORT INTO EVERYTHING THAT I DO.

I AM DILIGENT AND EFFICIENT.

I HAVE AFFECTIVE HABITS THAT HELP ME LEAD MY LIFE HEALTHILY.

I KNOW LIFE CAN AND WILL BE HARD. I WELCOME THE STRUGGLE BECAUSE I KNOW THE REWARD WILL OUTWEIGH THE TOUGH TIMES.

I HAVE HOPE THINGS WILL GET BETTER ONE DAY.

I KNOW HOW TO FIND THE HAPPINESS IN EVERYDAY THINGS.

I AM A SUCCESS STORY AND I CARRY MY WISDOM EVERYWHERE I GO.

I AM FULL OF HOPE AND JOY FOR THE FUTURE.

I KNOW MY FUTURE IS BRIGHT.

I KNOW I HAVE THE MEANS TO BE THE LEADER I WANT TO BE.

I AM A PROBLEM SOLVER, NOT A PROBLEM MAKER.

I WANT THE BEST FOR PEOPLE.

I AM PLEASED WITH THE PATH I HAVE TAKEN.

STRANGERS ARE FRIENDS.

I CAN EASILY COMMUNICATE WITH ANYONE.

IT'S EASY FOR ME TO MAKE FRIENDS.

I AM A HAPPY, OPTIMISTIC PERSON.

I AM CRITICAL WHEN I NEED TO BE.

I ANALYZE SITUATIONS AND LOGICALLY APPROACH
SOLUTIONS.

I TRY TO LOOK AT PROBLEMS FROM ALL
PERSPECTIVES.

I AM A LEAF IN THE WIND IN FALL. I BRING ABOUT
CHANGE.

I AM THE CALM BEFORE THE STORM'S EYE OPENS.
I AM THE STEADY THING.

I AM A WONDERFUL BEING.

I AM WORTHY OF SO MUCH.

I RESPECT OTHER PEOPLE'S OPINIONS, EVEN IF I DON'T SHARE IN THEM.

I AM A CHEERFUL PERSON.

I AM A LIVELY PERSON.

I AM ELATED TO BE ALIVE AT THIS MOMENT.

I AM DELIGHTED TO FACE EACH AND EVERY DAY.

I AM FULL OF BLISS.

I EMBRACE MYSELF FOR WHO I AM.

I EMBRACE OTHERS FOR WHO THEY ARE.

I AM MEANT TO BE HAPPY IN ALL THINGS.

I DESERVE THE BEST IN LIFE.

I DESERVE TO HOPE FOR BETTER THINGS, KNOWING I AM WORTHY OF THE BEST IN LIFE IS WHAT KEEPS ME GOING.

I AM NOT AFRAID, BECAUSE I TAKE LIFE IN STRIDE.

I HAVE MORE FIGURED OUT THAN I DID YESTERDAY, AND THAT KEEPS ME GOING.

I AM CONSTANTLY ADDING TO THE ARSENAL OF THINGS I HAVE LEARNED.

I GROW FROM THE THINGS I GO THROUGH.

I AM AN ACTIVE LISTENER.

I AM A GREAT STORYTELLER.

I TELL STORIES BECAUSE I KNOW THEY CAN RELATE TO SOMEONE.

I UNDERSTAND THE IMPORTANCE OF A TRUE, GENUINE CONNECTION.

I SEEK TO LEARN FROM THOSE AROUND ME THAT HAVE STORIES TO TELL.

I HELP UPLIFT OTHER VOICES.

I AM DESERVING OF THE SAME GENUINE CARE I GIVE TO OTHERS.

I LEAD MY LIFE IN LOVE.

I LEAD MY LIFE IN TRUTH.

I TELL MY TRUTH, SO OTHERS MIGHT BE INSPIRED TO DO THE SAME.

I TELL MY STORY TO THOSE WILLING TO HEAR.

I HAVE STORIES WORTH TELLING.

I KNOW SOMEONE CAN LEARN FROM THE THINGS I HAVE ACCOMPLISHED.

I KNOW SOMEONE CAN LEARN FROM THE THINGS I HAVE BEEN THROUGH.

I HAVE FAITH IN THE GOODNESS IN PEOPLE.

I KNOW I CAN RELY ON PEOPLE IN MY LIFE TO HELP WHEN I'M IN NEED.

I CHOOSE NOT TO WORRY ABOUT THE THINGS THAT ARE OUT OF MY CONTROL.

I CHOOSE TO LET THINGS "BE."

I HAVE NO DOUBT THINGS ARE GOING TO GET BETTER
FOR ME.

I HAVE HOPE TOMORROW WILL BE A SLIGHTER BETTER
DAY THAN THE ONE BEFORE AND SO ON.

I TRUST IN THE PROCESS OF THINGS.

I SEE THINGS THROUGH AND WAIT WHEN NECESSARY.

I AM FULL OF HOPE FOR THE NEXT YEAR AND THE
POSITIVE CHANGE IN STORE.

I AM A BEING THAT RADIATES
CONFIDENCE,
LOVE,
AND LIGHT
IN ALL THINGS I DO.

I AM INTENTIONAL ABOUT EVERYTHING I DO.

I BELONG IN THE SPACES I OCCUPY.

I KNOW THAT THERE ARE SOME THINGS I MIGHT NEVER BE ABLE TO CHANGE.
I'M OK WITH THAT.

I KNOW THERE IS SO MUCH I DO NOT KNOW.

I HAVE THE COURAGE TO SEEK OUT NEW DATA OR STATISTICS THAT MIGHT GO AGAINST MY VIEWPOINT.

I AM WILLING TO OPEN MY EYES TO NEW IDEAS, GOALS, AND DREAMS.

I AM NOT "SET" IN MY WAYS.

I AM ALWAYS OPEN TO CHANGE.

THINGS MIGHT BE HARD FOR A WHILE, BUT THINGS WILL TURN UP.

I AM A SONG SUNG IN TUNE TO A RHYTHM OF MY OWN.

I KNOW MY DREAMS ARE POSSIBLE; AND PROBABLE.

I CAN MANIFEST MY DREAMS, AND PUT IN THE WORK
TO MAKE THEM HAPPEN.

I KNOW THAT TO DO WELL I HAVE TO CHANGE MY BAD
MINDSET.

I DON'T HOLD ON TO NEGATIVE THINGS— I KNOW THEY
HOLD ME BACK.

I DON'T HOLD NEGATIVE THOUGHTS.

I TRY TO THINK POSITIVELY AS OFTEN AS I CAN.

I HAVE MORE THINGS FIGURED OUT THAN I DON'T.

I CHOOSE TO SMILE EVEN WHEN IT'S HARD.

I AM POWERFUL AND FULFILLED.

I CHOOSE TO BE THE BEST VERSION OF MYSELF
EVERY DAY.

I CHOOSE LOVE.

I CHOOSE WARMTH AND KINDNESS.

I DESERVE KINDNESS.

NOTHING IS TOO DIFFICULT.

NOTHING IS ENTIRELY IMPOSSIBLE.

BE YOUR OWN DEFINITION OF AMAZING.

MAKE YOURSELF PROUD.

WHEN EVERYTHING IS OVER, YOU WILL BE GRATEFUL
FOR STAYING TRUE TO YOURSELF.

YOU SHOULD BE PROUD OF THE LIFE YOU LEAD.

I CANNOT BE SHAKEN; I AM STEADY AND STRONG.

I FIND SOMETHING TO BE THANKFUL FOR EVERY DAY.

THE TREES GIVE ME AIR TO BREATHE.

I AM THANKFUL FOR THE EARTH IN SO MANY WAYS.

I BREATHE IN THE WORRIES, AND THE CONFLICTS, AND
EXHALE TO LET THEM GO.

SOMETIMES IT IS AS EASY AS LETTING GO.

STOP HOLDING YOURSELF BACK.

SOMETIMES ALL IT TAKES TO MAKE SOMEONE'S DAY IS
TO SMILE BACK.

TELL SOMEONE YOU LOVE THEIR SMILE TODAY.

I HAVE GRATITUDE FOR EVERYONE THAT HAS HELPED
ME ALONG THE WAY.

CHOOSE GOODNESS.

CHOOSE TO BRING PEACE TO SOMEONE'S
LIFE.

STOP AGONIZING OVER WHAT YOU DO NOT KNOW OR
UNDERSTAND.

JUST BE.

SURVIVE AND TRY TO THRIVE AS BEST AS
YOU CAN.

NOTHING IS AS HARD AS IT SEEMS WHEN
YOU HAVEN'T STARTED IT YET.

OBSTACLES ARE MEANT TO BE BLOWN OVER.

YOU HAVE THE POWER TO CHANGE THE WAY YOU
THINK ABOUT THINGS.

TRY HARDER.

STOP BEING NEGATIVE ABOUT EVERYTHING.

IT IS WAY TOO EASY TO GIVE INTO PESSIMISM.

WORK ON YOUR RELATIONSHIPS, THEY ARE WHAT
MATTER MOST IN THE LONG RUN.

DO NOT FORGET ABOUT WHERE YOU CAME FROM,
AND ALL THE EFFORT YOU HAVE PUT IN.

BE PROUD.

BE PROUD BECAUSE YOU ARE HERE.

YOU MADE IT THIS FAR.

EVERY GOAL YOU CRUSH IS A STEP IN THE RIGHT
DIRECTION— THIS INCLUDES JUST WAKING UP IN THE
MORNING.

I DO NOT LET LITTLE THINGS ANNOY ME.

I DO NOT LET RANDOM PEOPLE AFFECT ME.

I DO NOT LET THE SMALL THINGS GET TO ME.

I AM STRONG.

DIVINE BEINGS ARE NOT EASILY UNDERSTOOD.

EMBRACE YOUR UNIQUE SPIRIT.

STOP TRYING TO FIT IN.

STOP TRYING TO BE THE PERSON OTHERS WOULD
EASILY LIKE.

STOP TRYING TO BE ANYONE THAT IS NOT JUST THE
BEST VERSION OF YOU.

STOP GIVING IN TO PEER PRESSURE.

REALIZE YOU ARE BEAUTIFUL.

REALIZE YOU MAKE OTHERS WANT TO BE MORE
GENUINE VERSIONS OF THEMSELVES.

YOU MAKE THE WORLD A BETTER PLACE.

PEOPLE ADMIRE YOU.

PEOPLE ADMIRE THE WAY YOU LEAD YOUR LIFE.

PEOPLE ADMIRE THE THINGS YOU DO BECAUSE IT'S
THE "RIGHT THING TO DO."

PEOPLE ADMIRE YOU BECAUSE YOU LIVE FOR OTHER
PEOPLE'S HAPPINESS.

PEOPLE ADMIRE YOUR STRENGTH.

PEOPLE ADMIRE YOUR WORK ETHIC.

PEOPLE ADMIRE THE THINGS YOU DO FOR OTHERS.

SOMEONE IS GLAD TO HAVE YOU AS A FRIEND.

SOMEONE IS GLAD TO HAVE YOU IN THEIR FAMILY.

SOMEONE IS GLAD TO HAVE MET YOU IN PASSING.

YOU LEAVE A LASTING EFFECT ON PEOPLE.

YOU ARE NOT EASILY FORGETTABLE.

YOUR KINDNESS INSPIRES THE SAME IN OTHERS.

YOUR INDIVIDUALITY IS INSPIRING TO YOUNGER GIRLS.

YOU LIVE IN YOUR TRUTH AND THAT IS ALL THAT MATTERS.

YOU HAVE SO MUCH UNTAPPED POTENTIAL.

I KNOW THAT I AM WORTH THE EFFORT.

YOUR VOICE IS BEAUTIFUL, YOU SHOULD SING MORE.

YOU ARE SOMEONE'S EVERYTHING.

SOMEONE LOOKS AT YOU AND SEES THE BEST IN YOU.

SOMEONE LOOKS AT YOU AND SEES THE STARS IN YOUR EYES.

SOMEONE IS INSPIRED BY YOUR ESSENCE.

YOUR ENERGY IS VIBRANT.

YOUR ENERGY FILLS THE ROOM, IT IS GLEAMING WITH YOUR LIGHT.

YOU ARE THE "LIFE OF THE PARTY."

IN SO MANY WAYS, YOU ARE BEAUTIFULLY ONE OF A KIND.

YOU SHOULD BELIEVE IN YOURSELF MORE.
IT WOULD MAKE A DIFFERENCE.

USE YOUR VOICE FOR GOOD.

USE THE POWER WITHIN YOU TO OVERCOME
ADVERSITY.

YOU ARE SO WORTHY.

MORE THAN YOU WILL REALIZE, PEOPLE,
LOOK UP TO YOU.

PEOPLE TAKE STYLE INSPIRATION FROM YOU.

MAKE TODAY THE BEST DAY EVER, EVEN IF YOU'RE AT
HOME ALL DAY.

TAP INTO YOUR CREATIVE MIND FROM TIME TO TIME.

PAINT, LEARN A NEW LANGUAGE, READ; FEED YOUR
HUNGRY SOUL.

YOU ARE BEYOND AMAZING.

IF ONLY YOU KNEW WHAT OTHERS SEE IN YOU.

IF ONLY YOU COULD SEE THE WAY YOUR
LOVED ONES SEE YOU.

YOUR POTENTIAL IS AMAZING.

YOU CAN MAKE THE WORST TIMES, LESS PAINFUL.

YOU HAVE A LIGHT WITHIN YOU THAT BURNS BRIGHT;
SHOW THE WORLD WHAT YOU CAN
DO.

CHOOSE HAPPY. CHOOSE LOVE. CHOOSE THE
GOOD.

YOU ARE THE ROCKSTAR OF YOUR OWN SHOW.

YOU ARE THE MAIN CHARACTER.

GO THROUGH LIFE KNOWING YOU ARE THE MAIN
CHARACTER, NO ONE CAN PUT YOU DOWN.

I AM MADE OF SO MUCH CREATIVE ENERGY, THAT
JUST HAS YET TO BE TAPPED INTO.

STOP THINKING YOU ARE THE ONLY ONE BATTLING
THROUGH WHAT YOU ARE BATTLING THROUGH.

YOU ARE EVERYTHING YOU NEED.

YOU CAN TAP INTO YOUR CREATIVE MIND
WHEN NEED BE.

YOU KNOW YOU ARE THE ONLY PERSON YOU WILL
EVER NEED, BUT YOU LOVE PEOPLE.

YOU SET HEALTHY BOUNDARIES.

I AM CONSIDERATE.

I AM CONSIDERATE OF OTHERS 'TIME.

YOU PROTECT YOUR HEART AND MIND BY SETTING
BOUNDARIES WITH YOUR PARTNERS.

YOU ARE SOMEONE'S MUSE.

PROTECT YOUR HEART.

PROTECT YOUR LOVE.

BE PRESENT.

LIVE IN THE MOMENT.

YOU ARE LOVELY AND WONDERFULLY YOURSELF.

YOU MAKE ANYTHING YOU TOUCH YOUR OWN.

YOU HAVE A CREATIVE EYE THAT IS FULL OF
IMAGINATION.

I AM THE WRITER OF MY OWN STORY. NO ONE ELSE.

I KNOW I CAN DO ANYTHING.

I DO NOT NEED SOMEONE TO REMIND ME OF THAT.

I AM SELF-SUFFICIENT.

I AM MY OWN HELP.

I WANT TO MAKE MYSELF PROUD.

I AM EVERYTHING I WILL EVER NEED.

I HAVE THE DRIVE TO MAKE THE IMPOSSIBLE,
POSSIBLE.

I HAVE FAITH THAT NEXT YEAR WILL BE BETTER THAN
THIS.

I AM NOT EASILY DISAPPOINTED.

GREAT THINGS AWAIT ME.

I KNOW I WILL HAVE ABUNDANT OPPORTUNITIES IN THE FUTURE.

I KNOW THINGS WILL TURN UP FOR ME.

I AM SURE OF MYSELF.

I AM SURE OF MY GOALS AND ASPIRATIONS.

SUCCESS WILL FIND ME.

I AM A STRONG INDEPENDENT WOMAN.

I AM AT PEACE BECAUSE I KNOW WHERE I AM.

JUST TAKING A STEP IN THE DIRECTION OF MY DREAMS.

I AM THRILLED TO FACE THE DAY AHEAD.

I AM CONTENT WITH WHERE I AM RIGHT NOW.

I CAN SEE THE POSITIVE THINGS IN MY LIFE.

EVERY DAY IS A NEW CHANCE TO BE HAPPY.

I LOVE MYSELF AND WHO I AM YET TO BE.

I AM HAPPY WITH WHO I AM BECOMING.

I AM PROUD OF THE WOMAN I HAVE BECOME.

I AM SATISFIED WITH MY JOURNEY SO FAR.

I FEEL BLESSED AND THANKFUL FOR EVERYTHING I
HAVE RECEIVED IN LIFE.

I WOULD CONSIDER MYSELF A JOLLY PERSON.

I AM FULFILLED IN MY WORK LIFE.

I AM AT EASE.

ONE OF MY GREATEST ASSETS IS MY CARING ATTITUDE.

I AM SPONTANEOUS AND OPEN TO ADVENTURE.

I WANT TO EXPLORE.

I AM A LAID-BACK PERSON.

I KNOW I AM FLEXIBLE AND EASILY ADAPTABLE.

WHEN I CAN, I CHOOSE TO SPEND MY TIME WISELY ON THE THINGS THAT MATTER THE MOST TO ME.

I CHOOSE POSITIVITY.

I CHOOSE LOVE.

PROSPERITY AWAITS ME.

GOOD THINGS ARE COMING TO ME.

I WILL RECEIVE MORE THAN I EVER IMAGINED.

I DON'T HAVE UNREALISTIC STANDARDS.

I LIVE HAPPILY.

LIFE ISN'T BORING.

LEANING INTO THE GOOD.

LEANING INTO LOVE.

LEANING INTO THE LIGHT.

LEAN INTO THE JOY AND LET IT GUIDE YOU.
I LIVE WITH INTENTION.

I HAVE GOOD LUCK.

I DON'T HAVE TO WONDER ABOUT IF FATE LOOKS AT ME FONDLY.

I HAVE GREAT KARMA.

I AM FORTUNATE TO HAVE RECEIVED ALL THE THINGS I HAVE.

I AM THRILLED TO BE ME.

I AM SKILLFUL.

WHEN THINGS GET HARD, I DON'T GIVE UP.

WHEN THINGS BECOME UNMANAGEABLE, I TAKE A BREATH AND COOL-OFF.

TAKE EACH DAY IN STRIDE.

MAKE EVERYDAY A NEW REASON TO BE HAPPY.

THE SUN IS BRIGHT TODAY. TAKE IT IN.

EVERYTHING IS GOING TO BE OK.

TRUST THE PROCESS OF LIFE.

CHOOSE TO BE HAPPY EVEN WHEN IT'S HARD.

KNOW YOUR WORTH. LEAD BY THAT.

BE HONEST AND KIND. IT WILL TAKE YOU PLACES.

MAKE TODAY A GREAT DAY.

I AM LOVELY AS I AM.

LOOK IN THE MIRROR AND TELL YOURSELF
YOU ARE A QUEEN.

THERE IS NOTHING LIKE LOVE. TELL THE PEOPLE YOU
LOVE THAT YOU LOVE THEM.

I HAVE SO MUCH TO OFFER.

I AM AN ASSET TO ANY TEAM.

I HAVE THINGS FIGURED OUT.

I KNOW HOW TO CALM MYSELF.

TODAY COULD BE YOUR BEST DAY YET.

I HAVE EVERYTHING THAT I WILL EVER NEED.

EVEN IF THE DAY IS CLOUDY, THE SUN STILL MIGHT PEAK OUT.

STOP SEEING THE NEW DAY AS DULL— MAKE EVERY MOMENT AS EXCITING AS THE ONE PREVIOUS.

I AM POWERFUL AND STRONG.

I AM AT PEACE WITH MYSELF.

I AM CONTENT.

I AM STRONG AND DIFFICULT TO BREAK.

I WON'T WORRY ABOUT THE THINGS I CAN NOT CHANGE.

I KNOW HOW SKILLED I AM.

I DON'T LET IMPOSTER SYNDROME GET TO ME.

I KNOW MY ACCOMPLISHMENTS.

I DESERVE THE THINGS COMING TO ME.

I AM A WILD SOUL.

I HAVE A COURAGEOUS HEART.

I HAVE A WILD HEART THAT LOVES DEEPLY.
I HAVE A PURPOSE.

I CAN ACTUALIZE THE GOALS I HOLD MYSELF TO.
CONNECT WITH NATURE.

TAKE A WALK AND BREATHE IN DEEPLY.
I AM MAGNIFICENT.

I AM AS STRONG AS THE WIND DURING A WINTERS STORM.

I KNOW I AM CAPABLE.

I DO NOT NEED MALE VALIDATION.

I DO NOT NEED THE VALIDATION OF OTHERS.

I DO NOT NEED THE VALIDATION OF OTHERS TO FEEL WORTHY OR CAPABLE.

I AM GREAT.

I DO GREAT THINGS FOR OTHERS.

I CAN WITHSTAND ADVERSITY AND COME OUT STRONGER.

EVERYTHING I'M DOING RIGHT NOW IS ENOUGH.

I DO NOT NEED TO BE DOING MORE THAN I ALREADY AM TO BE OK.

I DON'T NEED TO OVERACHIEVE TO FEEL FULFILLED.

I GIVE OTHERS SUPPORT WHEN THEY NEED IT.

I HAVE EVERYTHING I NEED WITHIN ME.

I AM STRENGTH METASTASIZED.

I AM A BEAUTIFUL BEING.

I LOVE DEEPLY.

I AM ENOUGH AS I AM.

I AM A WORTHY BEING.

I AM BEAUTIFUL AT THE AGE I AM NOW.

I AM ONLY GOING TO GET BETTER WITH TIME.

I AM ONLY AS GREAT AS I ALLOW MYSELF TO BE.

I AM AMAZINGLY UNIQUE AND ONE OF A KIND.

I HAVE SO MUCH TO BRING TO THE TABLE.

I DON'T LET THINGS GET TO ME.

I HAVE THE STRENGTH I NEED INSIDE OF ME.

I AM COURAGEOUS.

I GIVE OTHERS SECOND CHANCES, WHY NOT GIVE
THAT TO MYSELF?

I AM FULL OF LOVE FOR THE EARTH AND NATURE.

I FEEL AT PEACE WITH MY JOURNEY.

I AM DETERMINED.

I WILL DO THE RIGHT THINGS.

I HAVE FAITH IN MYSELF.

I AM MY OWN PERSON.

I AM GRATEFUL FOR ALL I KNOW, AND I SEEK TO
BROADEN MY HORIZONS.

I AM BLOSSOMING LIKE THE FLOWERS.

MY MIND IS STRONG.

MY HEART IS STRONG.

TODAY IS FULL OF POSSIBILITIES.

EVERY DAY CAN'T LOOK LIKE OUR BEST DAYS.

EMBRACE THE PROCESS.

I AM GREAT.

I AM THE GOAT.

LET'S FACE TODAY WITH A SMILE.

YOU ONLY LIVE ONCE.

SEARCH FOR THE LIGHT AT THE END OF YOUR TUNNELS.

KNOW YOU ARE NOT FAR FROM HAPPINESS.

HAPPINESS IS JUST AROUND THE CORNER.

SUCCESS IS JUST AROUND THE CORNER.

FERTILITY IS JUST AROUND THE CORNER FOR YOU.

FINANCIAL FREEDOM IS JUST AROUND THE CORNER.

PERSONAL GROWTH IS JUST AROUND THE CORNER.

ACCEPTANCE IS JUST AROUND THE CORNER.

LOVE IS JUST AROUND THE CORNER.

LIVE HEALTHY.

LOYAL FRIENDSHIP IS JUST AROUND THE CORNER.

PLATONIC SOULMATES ARE IN YOUR FUTURE.

OPPORTUNITY IS JUST AROUND THE CORNER.

A RAISE IS IN THE CARDS FOR ME.

I CAN SEE MYSELF IN THE JOB I'M IN FOR A LONG TIME.

MY CAREER IS REWARDING.

I DON'T NEED ANY MATERIAL THING TO BE HAPPY.

MY HAPPINESS COMES FROM WITHIN. TOMORROW IS
A DIFFERENT DAY.

NEXT WEEK IS A NEW WEEK.

NEXT YEAR IS A YEAR TO START ANEW.

IT'S OK TO BE UNSURE OF YOURSELF. EMBRACE
NEWNESS.

TRY NEW THINGS.

FAIL. OFTEN. IT WILL TEACH YOU SOMETHING.

IT'S OK TO BE UNSURE OF WHERE YOU ARE GOING
AND WHAT YOU WANT TO DO.

LIVE AND LOVE IN THE FREEDOM OF SELF-
ACCEPTANCE.

CHOOSE SIMPLE JOYS.

BE MINIMALISTIC.

KNOW YOU ARE ENOUGH FOR SOMEONE.

SOMEONE IS GOING TO LOOK AT YOU AND LIGHT UP
WHEN THEY DO.

YOU ARE MAGICAL AND DIVINE.

YOU ARE A BEAUTIFUL SOUL.

PEOPLE ARE HAPPIER AND MORE AT PEACE IN YOUR
COMPANY.

LAUGH OFTEN.

DON'T TAKE YOURSELF SO SERIOUSLY.

BE SILLY AND HAVE FUN.

YOU ARE ONLY AS YOUNG AS YOU ARE RIGHT NOW.
BE YOUNG.

DO THE THINGS YOU NEVER IMAGINED YOURSELF
DOING.

TRY NEW HOBBIES, TAKE UP NEW SKILLS.

BE A LIFELONG LEARNER AND AVID READER.

KNOW THERE ARE LIMITS TO YOUR ABILITIES BUT THAT
YOU GIVE YOUR ALL IN EVERYTHING YOU DO.

LOOK BACK AT YOUR JOURNEY WITH GRATITUDE.

I AM EXTRAORDINARY.

I AM AMAZING.

I STAY CURIOUS.

I AM OUTSTANDING.

I AM PHENOMENAL.

MY SKILLS ARE UNPARALLELED.

I AM RARE.

AWESOME IS MY DEFAULT.

AMAZING IS MY DEFAULT.

STRONG IS MY DEFAULT.

I AM WONDERFUL.

WONDERFUL IS MY DEFAULT.

I AM STRENGTH INCARNATE. NOTHING HOLDS
ME BACK.

I AM THE CREATOR OF MY DESTINY. I AM
ALLURING.

I AM MARVELOUS.

I AM SPLENDID.

I AM CHARMING.

I AM GRACEFUL.

I AM FULL OF GRACE.

I AM A DELIGHT TO BE AROUND.

I AM LOVELY AS I AM.

I AM SWEET.

I AM FASCINATING.

I AM RAVISHING.

I AM ELEGANT.

I AM CUTE.

I AM NICE.

I AM INTERESTING.

MY CHARMS ARE ENCHANTING.

I CAN DO MOST THINGS I TRY.

MY BODY IS A VESSEL FOR MY INNER STRENGTH.

MY BODY IS A VESSEL FOR MY WONDERFULNESS.

MY BODY IS A VESSEL FOR MY AMAZINGNESS.

MY BODY IS A VESSEL FOR MY AWESOMENESS.

I ACKNOWLEDGE THAT I AM ENOUGH.

I ACKNOWLEDGE HOW STRONG I AM.

I ACKNOWLEDGE MY ABILITIES.

I ACKNOWLEDGE MY SKILLS AND GREAT QUALITIES.

I ACKNOWLEDGE THERE IS SO MUCH I HAVE LEFT TO LEARN.

I ACKNOWLEDGE I AM WORTHY.

I DESERVE THE GOOD THINGS IN LIFE.

I TAKE TIME FOR MYSELF.

I ACKNOWLEDGE I HAVE SO MUCH GROWING TO DO.

I ACKNOWLEDGE MY DREAMS ARE LIMITLESS.

MY DREAMS ARE LIMITLESS.

DREAM BIG.

SHOOT FOR THE STARS.

STOP GETTING IN YOUR OWN WAY.

BE THE BEST VERSION OF YOURSELF, YOU CAN BE.

ATTRACT GREAT ENERGY.

KNOW YOU ARE DOING THE RIGHT THINGS.

I LIKE MYSELF.

I LIKE WHO I AM BECOMING.

I UNDERSTAND THIS IS JUST ONE SMALL PART OF MY JOURNEY. THINGS WILL CHANGE.

I CAN ATTRACT THE ENERGY I NEED IN MY LIFE.

I CAN ATTRACT GREAT THINGS.

I CAN ATTRACT GREAT VIBES.

I CAN ATTRACT LOVE.

I CAN ATTRACT LAUGHTER.

I CAN MANIFEST THE REALITY I WISH TO HAVE.

I AM GRATEFUL FOR THE BODY I HAVE.

I AM GRATEFUL FOR THE BODY I CALL HOME.

MY BODY IS MY TEMPLE.

I CHOOSE MYSELF.

I CHOOSE LOVE.

I DO ENOUGH.

I AM ENOUGH.

I AM FEARLESS.

I AM MUTI-TALENTED.

MY BODY DESERVES REST.

I APPRECIATE MYSELF.

I APPRECIATE MY BODY.

I APPRECIATE MY MIND.

I APPRECIATE MY FAMILY AND LOVED ONES.

I APPRECIATE THE PEOPLE WHO CARE ABOUT ME.

I WILL STOP COMPARING MYSELF TO OTHERS. I AM
MORE THAN ENOUGH.

I WILL LOVE MYSELF FOR EVERYTHING THAT MAKES
ME, ME.

I WILL STOP LOOKING DOWN ON MYSELF.

I WILL STOP CRITICIZING MYSELF.

I AM SAFE.

I AM DOING AS BEST AS I CAN BE.

I AM WELL.

DO YOUR BEST ALWAYS AND YOU WON'T REGRET IT.

I WILL LET GO OF WORRIES THAT ARE OUTSIDE OF MY
CONTROL.

I AM IN CHARGE OF MY LIFE.

I DETERMINE THE PATH I FOLLOW.

I WILL BE THE CHOOSER OF MY DESTINY.

FATE WILL HAVE LITTLE TO DO WITH WHERE I END UP.

I AM MEANINGFUL.

I DO THINGS IN MEANING.

I DO THINGS WITH PURPOSE.

I AM DEFINED BY MY CONFIDENCE.

I KNOW WHO I AM.

I KNOW MY STRENGTHS AND MY WEAKNESSES.

I CREATE MY HAPPINESS.

I DON'T LIVE TO IMPRESS OTHERS.

I DON'T THRIVE OFF DRAMA.

I DON'T NEED TO IMPRESS OTHERS TO FEEL
VALIDATED.

I CAN CHANGE MYSELF.

I HAVE ALWAYS BEEN ENOUGH.

I AM IN CONTROL OF THE THINGS WITHIN MY CONTROL.

I DON'T WORRY ABOUT THE THINGS I CANNOT CHANGE OR FIX.

I DESERVE PLEASURE.

I DESERVE BLISS AND LOVE.

I CAN MAKE MISTAKES.

I AM ONLY HUMAN.

SLEEP COMES EASY TO ME.

I HAVE POTENTIAL.

LIKE AN UN-SHINED GEM, I WILL SPARKLE ONE DAY.

MY POTENTIAL IS LIMITLESS.

CAREER CHANGES AREN'T BAD.

A FRESH START IS SOMETHING I SEARCH FOR.

I LIKE TO KEEP THINGS NEW AND EVER- CHANGING IN MY LIFE.

I'M NOT A FAN OF THE BORING,

MY DESTINY IS ALREADY WRITTEN.

I HAVE HOPE FOR THE FUTURE.

I BELIEVE IN MYSELF.

I KNOW I WILL MAKE IT.

IT'S OK TO BE SAD.

IT'S OK TO NOT FEEL CONTENT SOMETIMES. T

RY TO SEE THE GOOD IN THINGS.

TRY TO SEE THE GOOD IN PEOPLE.

STOP LOOKING AT ONLY THE NEGATIVE.

I ASSERT MY RIGHT TO MESS UP.

I AM DOING MY BEST.

I AM DOING MY BEST AND THAT IS ALL I CAN DO.

I AM DOING MY BEST AND THAT IS ENOUGH.

MAKE OPPORTUNITIES FOR YOURSELF.

SEEK KNOWLEDGE.

SEEK OPPORTUNITY.

I HAVE BECOME THE WOMAN I HOPED TO BE.

I AM DIVINE.

I AM DIVINELY FEMININE.

I LIVE IN ACCORDANCE WITH MY VALUES.

I LIVE FOR MYSELF.

I AM WHOLE.

I AM NOT MISSING ANYTHING.

CHANGE YOUR THOUGHTS AND CHANGE YOUR LIFE.

I AM POWERFUL.

I HAVE INFINITE STRENGTH.

I GIVE MYSELF A BREAK SOMETIMES.

I TAKE IT EASY ON MYSELF.

I OFTEN SURPASS MY EXPECTATIONS FOR MYSELF.

I OFTEN SURPASS OTHERS' EXPECTATIONS.

I OFTEN SURPASS OTHERS' EXPECTATIONS OF ME.

I WILL BE PRESENT IN EACH MOMENT.

TODAY WILL BE GREAT.

TOMORROW WILL BE EVEN BETTER.

I AM BEAUTIFUL.

I AM THE PICTURE OF BEAUTY.

AS I AM, I AM WHOLE.

AS I AM, I AM ENOUGH.

AS I AM, I AM WORTHY.

AS I AM, I AM GLORIOUS.

AS I AM, I AM AWESOME.

AS I AM, I AM CONTENT.

AS I AM, I AM BEAUTIFUL.

AS I AM, I AM GORGEOUS.

AS I AM, I AM INTELLIGENT AND KIND.

I HAVE ACCEPTED MYSELF FOR MY FLAWS AND
EVERYTHING I AM.

I ATTRACT OPPORTUNITY.

I ATTRACT THE BEST THINGS LIFE HAS TO OFFER.

I AM INSPIRED.

I AM INSPIRED TO TRY MY BEST.

I AM INSPIRED TO DO MORE THAN WHAT IS EXPECTED OF ME.

I AM INSPIRED TO TRY HARDER.

I AM INSPIRED TO MAKE POSITIVE CHOICES IN MY LIFE.

I TAKE CARE OF MY HEALTH AND PAY ATTENTION TO MY EMOTIONS.

I AM IN TUNE WITH MY EMOTIONS.

I KNOW WHEN TO WALK AWAY.

I KNOW WHEN SOMETHING IS TOO MUCH FOR ME.

YOU ARE SO MUCH MORE THAN YOU ARE WILLING TO BELIEVE.

YOU ARE WONDERFULLY UNIQUE.

YOU ARE SO BEAUTIFUL.

YOU HAVE THE POWER TO FIX THE THINGS THAT
HAVE HELD YOU BACK.

OVERCOME THE IMPOSSIBLE.

I AM A BORN LEADER.

I AM RADIANT.

I AM WHOLLY MYSELF.

I CHOOSE KINDNESS.

I WILL SUCCEED IN MY ENDEAVORS.

I HOLD MYSELF TO GET HEIGHTS.

I WILL NOT FALL EASILY.

I WILL NOT FALL FOR OTHERS' LIES.

I CHOOSE TO LIVE DRAMA FREE.

I TAKE HEALTHY BREAKS FROM SOCIAL MEDIA.

I FOCUS ON THE THINGS I CAN CHANGE.

I FOCUS ON FIXING PROBLEMS.

I AM A PROBLEM SOLVER.

RADIATE CONFIDENCE.

RADIATE WHOLESOME ENERGY.

RADIATE LOVE.

RADIATE KIND ENERGY.

RADIATE GENEROUS ENERGY.

RADIATE AWESOMELY.

I AM A QUALITY PERSON.

I CAN AND WILL DO INCREDIBLE THINGS.

I'M FOCUSED ON MY GOALS AND ASPIRATIONS.

I LOVE AND RECEIVE LOVE IN RETURN.

MY RESOURCES ARE PLENTIFUL.

MY LIFE IS PLENTIFUL.

I SUPPORT MY BEST SELF.

I AM LEARNING HOW TO BE BETTER EVERY DAY.

I AM MY OWN MUSE.

I CAN HEAL MY OWN WOUNDS.

I CAN WORK ON MY INNER ISSUES AND FIX WHAT IS
BROKEN.

I CAN CONTROL MY THOUGHTS AND THE EMOTIONS
THAT FLOW THROUGH ME.

I AM MORE PRODUCTIVE EACH DAY.

EVERYTHING THAT IS MEANT TO BE, WILL BE.

I AM WHOLE AND ENOUGH.

I AM GRATEFUL FOR EVERY LITTLE THING.

I CAN RELAX AND LET LOOSE.

I IMAGINE A BETTER WORLD.

I STRIVE TO BE A GREAT HUMAN.

I SPEAK THE THINGS I WANT INTO EXISTENCE.

I CHOOSE NOT TO OVERTHINK.

WHEN I LIE IN BED, I DON'T WORRY ABOUT WHAT WAS
OR COULD BE.

I AM AT PEACE.

I FEEL PEACEFUL.

I KNOW I AM WHERE I AM SUPPOSED TO BE. THE THRILL
OF LIFE IS ALIVE.

I TAKE THINGS ONE STEP AT A TIME.

I DO NOT OVERDO MYSELF.

I DO WHAT IS NECESSARY. NOTHING MORE OR LESS.

I USE MY VOICE.

I TELL MY STORY FOR PEOPLE TO HEAR.

I AM WORTHY OF BEING LISTENED TO.

I GIVE GREAT ADVICE.

TODAY COULD BE WHAT DREAMS ARE MADE OF.

MAKE YOUR LIFE A LIVING DREAM.

I KNOW I CAN'T FIX EVERYTHING. I DON'T TRY TO.

I KNOW I CAN'T FIX PEOPLE. BUT I CAN LEND A HAND IN
SUPPORT.

I LEND MY FRIENDS HELPING HANDS.

I AM AWARE OF MY OWN BEAUTY.

I AM FULL OF KINDNESS FOR OTHERS.

I LOVE ANIMALS.

ANIMALS LOVE ME.

YOU ARE MAGIC.

YOU ARE MAGICAL.

YOU ARE ART.

YOU ARE BRAINS.

YOU ARE WIT.

YOU ARE THE DEFINITION OF BEAUTY.

YOU ARE THE DEFINITION OF KINDNESS.

YOU ARE THE DEFINITION OF SUNSHINE.

YOU ARE THE DEFINITION OF WARMTH.

YOU ARE THE DEFINITION OF JOY.

YOU ARE THE MANIFESTATION OF YOUR OWN DREAMS.

YOU ARE THE MANIFESTATION OF THE REALITY YOU CHOOSE FOR YOURSELF.

YOU ARE MUSIC TO SOMEONE'S SOUL.

YOUR SOUL SONG IS FULL OF PASSION AND JOY.

YOU ARE A CREATIVE BEING.

NOTHING CAN STOP YOU FROM ATTAINING GREATNESS.

YOU HAVE ALL YOU NEED WITHIN YOU. DREAM BIG AND SHOOT FOR THE BIGGEST STARS.

I CAN CHANNEL MY CREATIVITY.

I HAVE MEANINGFUL IDEAS.

MY IDEAS ARE WORTH SHARING.

MY CREATIVITY IS UNIQUE.

BE PRODUCTIVE IN THE THINGS YOU LOVE TO DO.

DO WHAT YOU WANT, OR YOU'LL BE STUCK DOING
WHAT OTHERS WANT YOU TO DO.

I AM JOY.

I AM AT PEACE.

I AM SILLY.

I AM KIND.

TODAY IS MY DAY.

I KNOW THE WORLD DOES NOT REVOLVE AROUND ME.

I AM POSITIVE.

THINK POSITIVE.

CHANGE YOUR POV ON THINGS.

MY MIND IS A BEAUTIFUL ASSET.

I AM BRAVE.

I STAND UP FOR OTHERS.

I HAVE MY FRIENDS' BACKS.

I LEAD THROUGH EXAMPLE.

I HAVE THE TOOLS TO SUCCEED WITHIN ME.

MY FUTURE IS BRIGHT.

I LET THE BAD GO AND KEEP THE GOOD WITH ME.

I AM JOYFUL.

I AM THE PICTURE OF CALM.

RELAXATION IS PART OF MY DAILY ROUTINE.

I INVEST IN SELF-CARE.

I INVEST IN THE THINGS THAT MAKE ME HAPPY.

LIVE WITH PURPOSE.

♥ thank you for your purchase!

Tattoos can increase feelings of confidence and improve self-image. Some feel that their tattoos allow them to look more like who they feel on the inside. If you found any tattoo that you liked in this book, please consider sharing your artwork with us and others who may benefit from it.

Your support means the world to us!

leave a review ♥

Copyrights 2023 - All rights reserved

www.ingramcontent.com/pod-product-compliance
Lightning Source LLC
Chambersburg PA
CBHW060252030426
42335CB00014B/1662